Cancer
Gifts

Cancer Gifts

Lessons In Gratitude
Acceptance and Perseverance

by
Linda Kopec

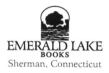

EMERALD LAKE
BOOKS
Sherman, Connecticut

DEDICATION

*In loving memory of my mother Alice
and all those who have lost their fight
with this disease called "cancer."*

*And in honor of my loving husband Dennis,
our two amazing daughters Jen and Emily,
and our son-in-law Ed, who has a heart of gold.*

CONTENTS

FOREWORD

This book is an inspiring memoir written by my mother, Linda Kopec, about surviving cancer, not once, but twice. It is a story of hope, determination, perseverance and faith. If cancer has touched your life in any way, I believe you will find yourself engaged from the very first paragraph.

Mom's determination through her cancer treatments repeated itself in her determination to write this book, which has been a collaboration in the works for eleven years. It's not just her perspective, though. It includes contributions written by her doctors, my father Dennis, and my sister Emily.

My mom's heartfelt down-to-earth stories also include important medical information and reflections on choices that had to be made.

This book is purposely written as short helpful chapters and is presented in chronological order. There are also captions with food for thought on every few pages called "Ringing the Bell" to help you explore the lessons that my mom learned on her own journey with cancer. The chapter titles are clever and witty, leaving you wanting to know more. For example, one chapter is called "The Lap Lady." What is that about, and who is the lap lady!?

Writing this book was a labor of love. My mom felt led to tell her story so that it might help someone else. Early readers have already expressed how it has helped them, and if you are holding this book, we hope it encourages you too.

My mom is always willing to talk with anyone who has questions or just to listen. When you have been through something like cancer, you become an asset and advocate for others as well. You never know when your life experiences may help someone else.

Chances are, you either know someone who has had cancer or have had it yourself. I don't know anyone who has not been changed by this disease. It doesn't even have to be cancer. It can be any medical situation. The principles and feelings are similar. You're overwhelmed with uncertainty and confusion, wanting answers, feeling scared, and just downright upset. It takes over your life and needs attention. These moments touch places in you and impact your life in ways you would never realize or think of. It is a journey. It really is. Just show up the best you can. Ask questions and take someone with you to be your support.

It is with deep love, gratitude and honor that I write this foreword for my mom Linda. She has been changed by cancer. We all are changed by cancer, and we are continually learning from this. Yet, she has shown such courage, strength and faith as she faced her cancer journey that she touched the lives of those around her. You would never know how hard it was for her. She carries herself with such a positive attitude, always moving forward, moving on to the next thing. She has taught me that life is meant to be lived. So, keep learning from experiences and moving forward.

To all the caregivers out there, make sure to be good to yourself. Eat well, drink water, get rest, and consider joining a support group. Whatever you do, make sure you have support. Cancer is too much for someone to go through on their own. One thing this book gets across is it takes a team effort on every level. Stuff you would never even think of. Be open to the experience. You never know what's next...

—Jen Kopec

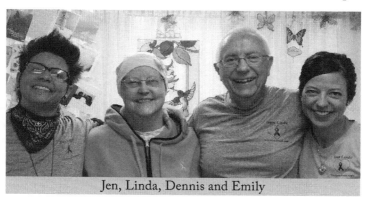

Jen, Linda, Dennis and Emily

INTRODUCTION

If you're picking up this book, you have probably been touched by cancer in some way. Perhaps a diagnosis was recently received by a friend, a family member, or even yourself. No one wants to hear the dreaded C-word. But when you do, it's natural to want to know what you are in for. More importantly, you are looking for hope. You want someone to tell you it's going to be alright, that there's a way through this diagnosis that leads to peace and happiness, if not full restoration to health.

I've been in your shoes, not once, but twice! So I can guess what you're feeling.

I was quietly living my life, working full-time and contentedly married to my husband, having raised two wonderful daughters together.

Then everything changed. Suddenly, I received my first cancer diagnosis, Stage 4 colon cancer, and my world was turned upside down.

I was scared. Not knowing what to expect. Not knowing if I would survive. Worrying how this would affect my husband and my children.

While I would find my way to being cancer-free again a year later, it wasn't without its challenges. That feeling of being afraid never quite left me as I navigated my way through the treatment process.

When I was diagnosed with Stage 3a breast cancer ten years later, I couldn't help but wonder, "Why me? I've already been through this before."

Being a completely different cancer, my treatment regimen was completely different too. While I had chemotherapy and surgery the first time, this time, I had chemo, surgery and radiation.

At first, when I kept wondering why I was going through this again, there was no answer. But over time, I became convinced that this was to serve as an inspiration of sorts.

I had a close-knit family and supportive healthcare team. But what about those cancer patients who don't have that or who don't know how to ask for what they need? Or who don't even know what they might want? And what about those caregivers who wish they knew how to be more helpful and supportive of a loved one facing cancer?

That is what inspired me to write this book. By sharing my story, my goal is that, as you take a ride on my emotional rollercoaster, you will see that there is hope among the fear and beauty among the ashes.

There are people who care about you and who want to see you healthy and well again. With their encouragement and care, you will become a stronger person. This experience will teach you more about yourself than you've ever known before. No matter what your particular journey entails, as time passes, there will be beauty in it.

May my story bring you hope as you make your journey and remind you that you are not alone.

A Very Unusual Day

It was a cold winter day in February 2005. The alarm clock went off, and it was time to get up for work. I showered, dressed, had a quick bite to eat, and was off to work. Traffic on the highway that day was moving along without any tie-ups or accidents. I was always glad to arrive at work safely and on time.

As I entered the building, I said "Good morning" to Kathy, our receptionist.

She replied, "Payroll checks have been delivered and are on your desk."

At that time, I worked as a payroll bookkeeper in a nursing home. As I was getting the checks in order for each department, I started having severe pain in my lower abdomen. *What was the matter with me?* My head was hot with fever. Maybe I was coming down with the flu. There was no way I could stay at work. I needed to go home.

Since I was feeling so poorly, I didn't feel up to driving myself home. My boss agreed to drive me. Then a friend offered to follow us in my car. It was so good to get home, but the pain was still severe. My husband Dennis was at work, and our daughters were grown and lived out of state. I was all alone and not sure what to do.

As I sat quietly, I began feeling worse. This was not good. I couldn't just sit there. What if I passed out? No one would know.

I had such an uneasy feeling that I decided the best thing for me to do was to call the doctor. I explained my pain to him, and he told me to come in right away. Since his office wasn't far from home, I felt confident I could drive myself there. I sure was glad my friend had driven my car home for me.

Still in pain, I arrived at his office. He greeted me as I opened the door. "Linda, come right into the examining room."

I was so glad I didn't need to wait. I explained my pain and told him where it hurt.

After the examination was over, he said it was not the flu. "Sounds like an attack of diverticulitis: here is a prescription for you. I want you to go home and rest for a few days, then come back next week to see me again."

The next week, I went back for my follow-up visit. I was feeling much better. It was such a relief to not have that pain anymore, but unexpectedly he strongly urged me to have a colonoscopy. He gave me the name of a doctor across the hall from his office. I felt better and was putting it off, but then I thought maybe there is something more going on and I just didn't know. I sure didn't want the pain to come back.

Finally, I got the courage to call and make the appointment. Because of my attack, I was given an appointment right away. I was considered an emergency case... "What?"

I wondered. "Why am I an emergency case? What is going on with me? What is wrong?"

Then I thought about my job. *How can I work if I have something seriously wrong?* There were so many thoughts going through my mind, and it seemed like my world was turning upside down.

It was February 23, 2005, when I first met Dr. Nkemakonam Ikekpeazu. I explained the pain I had had two weeks earlier.

After we talked a while he said, "We need to know for sure what caused the pain." He recommended I have a CT scan.

Now I was really scared. I didn't even know what a CT scan was.

On Friday, March 3, 2005, I had the CT scan. It was explained to me this is a computerized scan that combines a series of x-ray images taken from different angles around the body. It uses computer processing to create cross-sectional images of the bones, blood vessels and soft tissues inside the body.

The next day, Dr. Ikekpeazu called me and told me the results of the scan. He said, "You have an abscess on the outside of your colon, and it is quite serious. You need to have a drain put in very soon. I want you to go to the hospital on Monday, and we will do this right away."

I said okay, but really didn't understand what was going to be done. I was so surprised by the call that I didn't know what questions to ask and wasn't thinking clearly. Different thoughts were running through my mind. *Am I going to be all right? How serious is this?*

My husband is an accountant and, being the middle of tax season, Dennis was very busy. Since the doctor had made the procedure sound fairly routine, I took my friend Debbie up on her offer to take me so Dennis could go to work. So, on the following Monday, Debbie and I went to St. Raphael's Hospital. The procedure to attach the drain took about an hour.

When it was over, there was a tube about three feet long lying on my stomach that connected to a bag. The tube protruded from my groin to drain the abscess. The whole thing was very uncomfortable, and I was completely overwhelmed. I had no idea how I was going to manage getting up and moving around with all this paraphernalia to work around. I felt mortified and ready to cry, wondering how I was supposed to put my pants on with this tube hanging out of me.

The nurse saw how upset I was and offered to assist me. She secured the tube to my leg and helped me get dressed.

This was not what I expected when the doctor said he would put a drain in for the abscess. I hadn't been prepared for what it would be like and only knew that there was another CT scan taken during the procedure that was used for guiding the doctor's work.

I just wanted to go home and cry. Finally, we could leave the hospital, and I was glad to be home and in bed. What an exhausting day!

It wasn't until a few days later that I found the information online that I needed to understand the drain procedure. It explained that the

RINGING THE BELL

Have you ever been surprised by a lack of information? If so, how did it make you feel? During this cancer journey, be sure to ask questions. The more information you have, the better you'll be able to make important decisions about your treatment and care. And if you're feeling overwhelmed or aren't comfortable asking questions, appoint a trusted family member or friend to advocate for you.

surgeon uses a CT scan to locate the abscess. Then, it is drained using a needle. A small incision is made in the skin over the abscess and a thin plastic tube called a "drainage catheter" is attached. The catheter allows the abscess to drain into a bag and is usually left in place for a week.

At the time of my procedure, our house was undergoing construction. We were building a new kitchen and garage. The whole side of the house was open with just a plastic tarp covering it. It was the second week of March, and it was so cold.

When I got home from the hospital, our house felt like a wind tunnel. We called our daughter Emily to tell her how things went with the drain. I was in bed at the time, resting and trying to keep warm. As soon as we told her how cold the house was, she said right away, "Mom, you can't stay there in the cold. Come stay with me, so you will be warm."

Emily lives in upstate New York, a five-hour drive from where we live in Connecticut. It was decided Dennis would drive halfway, and Emily would drive the other half. So, Dennis got me settled in the car with a pillow and blanket and off we went to meet her.

By the time Emily and I arrived at her house, we were both so... so... tired. She put sheets and blankets on the couch in the TV room so I wouldn't need to climb the stairs to the bedrooms. It was hard to settle down from the long day.

I tried to process the day's events. The morning had started with going to the hospital with Debbie, having the CT scan, and getting the drain put in. After the procedure, I had the shock of seeing the long tube on my belly, the nurse helping me get dressed, and returning home with my instructions.

Finally, there was the five-hour car ride to Emily's house. I was so exhausted, I just wanted to cry.

The next day, Emily went to work. After she left, I called my boss and told him I was in New York dealing with this drain and couldn't come to work. My boss had no choice but to learn my payroll job since it was Tuesday, the payroll transmission day. Checks needed to be processed for the next week's payroll for 206 employees. After we made many phone calls back and forth from New York to Connecticut, the payroll was finally done. Another exhausting day!

While Emily was at work, I rested as best I could. I hated the drain and wanted it out. A foreign body could cause infection, which I sure didn't want to have happen. I also feared, if I moved the wrong way, it might come out on its own. Then I would be in big trouble. I definitely didn't want to go back to the hospital to have it put in again—let alone needing to go to a New York hospital. I needed a lot of patience.

On Wednesday and Thursday, it snowed all day. Upstate New York gets lots of lake-effect snow. It was lonesome while Emily was at work, but when she came home in the evening, I felt a little better.

Friday arrived, and it was time to go back home to Connecticut. I had an appointment with Dr. Ikekpeazu in the afternoon. I thought this would be the day the drain would come out. Emily helped me into the car, and we headed for Connecticut.

When we arrived at the doctor's office, the waiting room was filled with people. I was very weak and not feeling well at all. The drain was more than I could handle and was making me very emotional. I tried to hold back my tears, but sitting in the waiting room seemed to last forever.

When it was finally my turn to see the doctor, I thought, *Now he will take it out.* Instead, he explained to Emily and me how serious the abscess was and that I needed to keep the drain in another week. Not what I wanted to hear...

This can't be happening. I left the doctor's office ready to cry. There was nothing I could do.

Family Love

While I was in New York with Emily, the builders continued working on our house. They closed up the opening where the tarp was, so the house was much warmer. I was glad to be home.

When it was time for Emily to go back to her job in New York, we said goodbye with tears in our eyes. It is hard to live so far away from each other, but I was glad to be home with Dennis. We talked about all the things that happened during the past week. So much to process...

Talking with him helped me settle down, and I finally had a good night's sleep. The next morning Dennis left for work, and I continued to rest in bed.

Dr. Ikekpeazu called for a visiting nurse to check on me, which I was glad for since I was home alone. The nurse made me feel better and not so lonely. She checked the drain to make sure it was clean and the wound was okay.

By the third week in March, I needed another CT scan to see if the abscess had drained enough. This was now my third CT scan. I was so sure it had drained enough and would be taken out. But, no! The hospital doctor told me,

"It needs to drain more." That left me feeling so down. My spirit seemed lost.

At least, the visiting nurse was coming the next day and would come every day that week. She made me feel better and safe. Knowing that all was well with the drain and wound helped me to relax.

In the fourth week of March, it was time to go back to the hospital for the fourth CT scan to see if the abscess had drained enough. To my surprise, the doctor told me, "I think it's time to take out this drain." Shocked… I asked her to repeat what she just said. The drain had been in for a total of seventeen days. Finally, it was coming out. Thank God. This was the most traumatic experience I have ever had.

RINGING THE BELL

Sometimes, a "bad" experience can actually turn out to be the best thing that could have happened to us. Can you recall a time in your life when a painful or upsetting experience turned out to be just what you needed?

When the doctor was finished, I asked her to help me up from the operating table since I was still very weak. Dennis and Emily were in the waiting room. At last, I had good news. I walked into the waiting room with a big smile and a thumbs up, looked at the two of them, and said, "Let's go home!" They each smiled back at me, knowing that the drain was out. What a relief!

During all this time, my other daughter Jen was on the West Coast working. We kept in touch regularly by phone. A few days after the drain was taken out, Jen came back to Connecticut. It was so good to see her and spend time together. I told her, "As much as having the drain was such an emotional experience, it saved my life. If the abscess had burst, I might not have lived." I was blessed to have made it through. We hugged for a long time. We have always been a close family, but this brought us even closer.

I told Jen my next step was a colonoscopy and assured her, "Actually, I want the colonoscopy. I want to make sure there isn't anything else going on."

Jen was such a comfort to me. "Mom, you are going to be fine."

We had such a wonderful visit together, I didn't want it to end. But soon it was time for Jen to head to Cape Cod, Massachusetts, four hours away from home, since she was beginning a new job the following week.

MESSAGE FROM DR. DAWN KOPEL, GYNECOLOGIST

As an outpatient gynecologist, much of my day is spent on routine screening, examinations and problem-solving. The screening tests commonly performed for women include Pap smears and mammograms, the latter being done by radiology professionals. I generally adhere to the screening guidelines pretty closely, only occasionally adjusting them as needed based on patient situation and preference. In the end, it is an informed and joint decision.

When one of these screening tests come back as abnormal, there is often the angst associated with having to deliver unpleasant or potentially devastating news to a patient, combined with the patient's own fears and worries.

Moments like this demand honesty, clarity, compassion and continued support as she moves into the next phase of treatment. This is especially so if she is being transferred to another specialist or facility. And it is in these moments that I learn some of the greatest lessons my patients have to teach.

While I had already known Linda for a few years beginning with her colon cancer, her new diagnosis of breast cancer was a continuation of my education by way of her grace and positivity. She navigates life's difficulties by way of her profound faith, further buoyed by the profound love and devotion of her family and friends.

Linda received her care at Smilow Cancer Hospital at Yale New Haven, which we are lucky to have at our virtual doorstep. I have no doubt that having access to advanced care at a leading cancer center made a difference in Linda's prognosis, in addition to her positive outlook, attitude and faith.

I truly enjoy my profession in so many ways. I find the study and practice of medicine endlessly fascinating and relating to people as individuals similarly engaging. I love how being a doctor allows one to be a lifelong student as well as a practitioner. It is immensely gratifying to be part of patients' lives, to provide medical care, and to do my small part in educating my patients and relieving suffering when called upon to do so.

I commit myself to the welfare of my patients every day and am grateful for the opportunity to partake in their care. I am also grateful for the opportunity to share these thoughts with you.

A MUSTARD SEED

The colonoscopy was scheduled for the second week of April. Dennis and Emily took me to the Hamden Surgery Center, and Dr. Ikekpeazu began the procedure. Unfortunately, it could not be completed. I was still too swollen from the abscess. I would need another seven weeks to heal before we could try again.

Oh, no! That was not what I wanted to hear. My heart sank, and I thought, "It's been one problem after the next. When are these roadblocks going to stop?"

My next colonoscopy was scheduled for the end of May. By this time, the swelling was gone and Dr. Ikekpeazu was able to complete the procedure. Six polyps were found. He was able to remove five of them, but the sixth one was too large, which meant going back to the hospital for surgery.

I began to wonder, *Do I have the dreaded C-word?* It felt like a dark cloud was hanging over me, and it wouldn't go away.

During this time, I returned to work part-time. Since a payroll job is so timely and detailed, a temporary employee named Debbie was hired to assist me. I showed her all the things that needed to be done to keep up with my responsibilities. This would prepare her for when I was out of the office for the surgery.

Surgery day came on July 5, 2005, and I was ready to get it done and over with. My surgery was quite long, taking more than five hours. While I was in recovery, Dr. Ikekpeazu explained to Dennis, Jen and Emily that the surgery had not been easy to perform.

When he went in, Dr. Ikekpeazu found I had Stage 4 colon cancer, which had spread from my colon to my left ovary to my lymph nodes. He needed to remove 40% of my colon, the ovary, and thirty-six of the lymph nodes in that area of my body. This is why the surgery took so long,

Fortunate for me, only six of those lymph nodes were cancerous. But it meant I would need chemotherapy just in case any cancer cells remained.

Oh, no! I thought. *All this time, I had cancer and didn't know it.* Trying to process the last few months had my mind on overload. Thinking back to the day at work in pain, going to my doctor's office, meeting a new doctor, having a CT scan, the drain being put in for seventeen days, an unsuccessful colonoscopy, the second colonoscopy finding six polyps, surgery to take the largest polyp out, and now finding out I will need to go through chemotherapy.

Is my faith being tested? Because I am feeling as tiny as a mustard seed...

The kingdom of heaven is like a grain of mustard seed which a man took and sowed in his field; it is the smallest of all seeds, but when it has grown it is the greatest of shrubs and becomes a tree, so that the birds of the air come and make nests in its branches.

MATTHEW 13:31b-32, RSV

THE LAP LADY

There was no choice but to accept the reality that I had cancer. As I lay in my hospital bed, I thought of Dennis, Jen and Emily. They had been through so much with me, with much more to go. I felt badly that I was putting them through all of this.

In life, there is no way to predict what challenges will come our way. Each of us receives unexpected news throughout our life. This makes us look at things from a different perspective.

The night of the surgery, my nurse said she was going to get me up. She wanted me to walk from the bed to the door of my room. I thought she was crazy. My belly was sore, so she told me to hold a pillow against it as I got up from my bed. Surprisingly, it did help.

The next day she came to my room and said I needed to walk around the nurses' station. She told me, "This will give you some exercise and get your system moving." So again, I held the pillow against my belly and slowly got up from my bed. The nurse took my arm and walked with me around the nurses' station. I did alright, but was glad to return to my bed and get some rest.

A couple hours later, I got up again, but this time by myself. I held the pillow to my belly and started walking.

My nurse saw me and asked, "Do you want me to walk with you?"

I replied, "No, thank you. I think I can walk by myself." I did just fine, and it made me feel good to be independent.

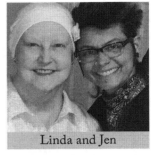
Linda and Jen

Each day, I was getting stronger and began walking two and three times around the nurses' station. They started to call me "The Lap Lady."

I recuperated in the hospital for six days before finally returning home.

CHEMOTHERAPY

The day came for me to go home. I was so excited. Beautiful flowers and cards were awaiting me there, sent by family members and friends to wish me well. It warmed my heart to be remembered by so many people. The best part though was being home with Dennis, Emily and Jen. I am so grateful for my wonderful family who helped me through this series of events.

On July 20, 2005, I met Dr. Vijay Chhabra, who became my oncologist. My husband and daughters were with me. We had a lot of questions about chemotherapy. Our conversation lasted an hour and a half.

Dr. Chhabra told us the surgery had removed all the cancer, but the chemo treatments would maximize the surgery's effectiveness. The treatments would take place

RINGING THE BELL

Everyone faces different circumstances as they take this journey. Some have family nearby that they're close to. Others don't. Having a support team you can count on is important. Who can you count on to be there when you need them? Do you have family who will be there for you? Or friends who are like family? Think about who you've been able to count on in the past and ask them to be on your team.

over six months. And then, of course, we learned about the side effects. I might have numbness in my hands and feet, fatigue or loss of appetite. I would especially need to avoid being exposed to the cold during the winter. The doctor told me I couldn't eat cold foods or drink water from the refrigerator since it would numb my mouth. While the numbness would potentially be uncomfortable, it could also be hazardous when eating or chewing.

Before I could have my chemotherapy treatments, I would need to have a port-a-cath, or "port," put in, which meant another trip to the hospital. I was glad Dr. Chhabra explained to me what the port was. A port-a-cath is a small device that consists of a port with a tube (or catheter) attached. The surgeon will make a small cut in the neck to access a vein. The catheter is then connected to the vein and the port is fitted into a space created under the skin in the upper chest.

He told me the chemo drugs would go through this port into my blood stream. By having it connected to a vein, I wouldn't need to be poked with a needle at each treatment since the port is always accessible for the nurses, both for drawing lab work as well as administering my treatments.

On August 2, 2005, the port was installed. I left the hospital and went directly to the oncology center for my first chemo treatment. Emily gave me a beautiful yellow rose with a card that read, "To represent your courage throughout."

Dennis, Jen, Emily and I arrived at the center very apprehensive. This would be my longest treatment (five hours) as the drugs would need to be given to me slowly through my port. My system would need time to adjust.

While we were there, a patient named George was having his treatment and could see how nervous we all were. He was so kind to us. He said, "Your body needs to adjust. It gets better as you go along." Those simple words gave us more comfort than he knew.

When the treatment was over for the day, I learned I would need to wear a pump. This was to be connected to my port so medication could continue to be administered. The pump was in a fanny pack that went around my waist. As it did its job, I could hear noises that assured me it was working.

RINGING THE BELL

Often when we're struggling, the best thing we can do to help ourselves is to help someone else. Even when you're not feeling well, words of encouragement, like George's to me, and a friendly smile go a long way toward brightening your day and someone else's!

Sleeping was a challenge. I was so afraid the line from the pump to the port might disconnect. Soon, I discovered that laying on my side with my arms stretched out in front of me helped.

The next day, I went back to the treatment center, and the pump was disconnected. The nurse started another treatment via the port for five hours. After this was finished, I was reconnected to the pump and had to wear it for another twenty-four hours.

On the third day, a nurse came to my house to disconnect the pump. This was the end of the first treatment. The whole process took forty-nine hours. I was so exhausted, it was hard to settle down. My mind raced as it tried to process the past three days and wondered what would happen between now and my next treatment in twelve to fourteen days.

Before each treatment, I needed to have blood work done to check my white and red blood cell levels. If they were too low, my treatment had to be delayed until the levels came back up.

On the bright side of all this, Emily took me to the movies after my treatment. During the week, we had the movie theater mostly to ourselves. I tried to avoid crowds for fear of germs because my immune system was low due to the chemo treatments. The movie took my mind off of the treatment and helped my body adjust to the chemo as I sat quietly watching.

Sometimes, we took a walk by the beach where I live. I love the fresh air, as it always makes me feel better and is so peaceful. Some days, I walked ten minutes and, other days, I walked thirty. It depended on my endurance at the time.

August 16, 2005, was the date for my second treatment. Dennis needed to go to work, so Emily traveled again from upstate New York to be with me so I wouldn't be alone at the treatment center. She brought me a card with a message of encouragement. "To represent your positive attitude and outlook." It came with two purple irises to represent my second treatment.

As my blood levels started to drop, I needed to go to the center Monday through Friday to get a Neupogen injection to boost my white blood cells and once a week for a Procrit injection to do the same for my red blood cells. I was beginning to feel like a pin cushion.

Emily stayed with me for the three days of the treatment, but then needed to return to her job in New York. Because I was so weak and didn't feel up to driving myself to get my injections, my sister Joan and my niece Amy volunteered to take me to the center.

Message from
Dr. Vijay Chhabra, Oncologist

I am a hematologist and oncologist at Oncology Hematology Care of CT, with specialties in cancer treatment and blood disorders.

As an oncologist, I was trained to treat many cancers. Linda had colon cancer in 2005 when I took care of treatments for her. Then in 2016, Linda was diagnosed with breast cancer and I took care of treatments for her again.

In addition to medical issues, I feel the most important factor in Linda's prognosis was her determination to be treated and face the disease.

For each patient, I follow standard protocol and my major source is the National Comprehensive Cancer Network.

However, as a person, I like to treat people and not the disease only. What I enjoy most about my profession is helping patients and seeing the smiles on their faces.

The advice I give a patient is to always remember that hope and determination are as important as any medical therapy. I can provide the treatment, but that's only part of the equation. They have to believe that the treatment is the right thing for them and be committed to seeing it through.

Everybody on this earth has their own journey to take. And medicine alone can only take them so far in their healing process. The rest is up to them.

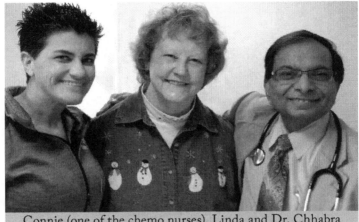
Connie (one of the chemo nurses), Linda and Dr. Chhabra

THE OUTINGS

Labor Day weekend was approaching, and Emily wanted to take Dennis and me to Niagara Falls in Canada. I felt up to going, but still needed my injections to keep my blood levels up for the next treatment. At my next visit, I told Dr. Chhabra about the trip and that I really wanted to go.

He said, "No problem." He called the pharmacy and ordered the needles for me. Then he showed Dennis how to give me the injection. Never did I think my husband would be giving me needles.

Niagara Falls was so beautiful, and it was such a wonderful trip. It truly was special family time.

My third treatment was September 7, 2005. My fatigue and tiredness increased, and I was starting to lose weight. I didn't have much of an appetite. One of the side effects of the chemo is a choking feeling, which caused me not to want to eat. I also had a metallic taste in my mouth, so food didn't taste good.

As I underwent the treatments, I tried to keep my days as normal as possible. I got up as if I was going to work, but instead I went out with Joan and Amy. On my good days, when I felt up to eating, we went out for lunch. They also took me to get my nails manicured. Having my nails look nice always makes me feel better.

Before my treatments started, I bought a wig. I wasn't sure if I would lose my hair, but wanted the wig just in case I needed it. It was very expensive. Now it was time to start using it. My hair was thinning (although not falling out). I was losing my eyebrows and eyelashes, and the days were getting colder.

To my disappointment, I didn't feel comfortable wearing the wig. I just didn't look like myself. With the colder weather, I needed to cover my head, face and hands. The cold was making me feel numb.

So, one day I went shopping with my sister Joan and my niece Amy. I tried on many different colors of hats, gloves and scarves to match. The hats looked much better than the wig and gave me some color as I was looking very pale. I felt more like myself that way, and the hats made me smile.

What a great shopping day!

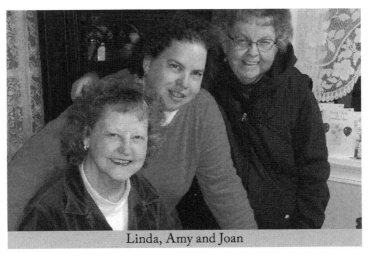

Linda, Amy and Joan

THE CARROT

As I received more treatments, different side effects appeared. My eyes became watery, the numbness in my hands increased, and I kept dropping things. One side effect I had to be very careful of was mouth sores. I was told to use salt and warm water every day as a precaution. Fortunately, I didn't have any sores.

My nails were starting to thin too, much like wax paper. My manicurist used a special polish, telling me, "This polish will help a little until the chemo treatments are over."

By the sixth treatment, I found myself so excited to be halfway through. Joan and Amy shared in my excitement. They each gave me a little gift to celebrate.

To my disappointment, I became sick to my stomach during the treatment, which needed to be stopped as a result. Another appointment had to be set up to repeat treatment number six. I was

RINGING THE BELL

Things rarely go according to plan. The sooner you accept that, the easier things will be for you. Develop your ability to adapt and be flexible, and find ways to reward yourself when you make it through something challenging. Rewards make all the difference!

so disappointed. I couldn't help thinking, "Why do I keep having setbacks?"

As the months went by Dennis, Jen and Emily started planning a trip to Disney World in Florida. They dangled this carrot in front of me to celebrate the end of my chemo treatments. It would be a time of family, love and life together.

January 3, 2006, was the day I was supposed to have my tenth treatment, but my platelets dropped so my treatment needed to be delayed a week. I felt weaker and had a lot of numbness in both my hands and feet. I still dropped things and had very little strength in my hands. My feet were sore, and I started losing my balance.

When I made it to treatment number eleven, Emily brought me eleven pink hyacinths with a card that read:

> *Dear Mom, for your acceptance of not "being in control" and letting Him take care of everything and trusting that it will all be taken care of... for you! Love, Em*

The day finally arrived for my twelfth treatment. This would be my last dose of chemo. It was February 13, 2006.

My friend George was at the center having his treatment. He asked me, "Linda, how are you doing?"

I smiled and told him, "It is my last one, George."

He was so happy for me. Two weeks later, I went back for a checkup and learned that George had passed away... I will always remember his words of encouragement that first day. George, may you rest in peace, my dear friend.

As the months went by, I thought of how far I had come. It took almost an entire year, with my family always by my side. They were with me through the up and down days of disappointments and feeling lost. They supported me through all the setbacks I faced. I have truly been blessed with a loving husband and two great daughters. I had been on this cancer journey a long time. But I wondered, "Is there a way I could share my experience with other people and bring them hope?" This question stayed with me even as I continued my treatments.

For treatment number twelve, Emily brought me a beautiful arrangement of twelve assorted pastel roses. The card I received from her to represent this treatment reads:

> *The last one. I know we thought this day would never get here. You have done amazing! You have gotten through these treatments so successfully and now are wanting to share your experience with others. You want to give others the hope, courage, encouragement and words of wisdom so they will be as successful as you have been. I love you, Emily.*

On February 15, 2006, my nurse Alice came to my home to disconnect the pump. This ended the last treatment. She was so happy for me.

Emily took pictures of us, smiling. This is the last time I would see Alice since I was finished with chemo. Amen. When I said goodbye to her, I thought of my mother. You see, my mother's name was Alice. (I miss you, Mom.)

On March 19, 2006, my family and I set out for Disney World to celebrate life. This was the trip I had been looking forward to during all the months of chemo. It was the most wonderful family week of celebrating life and love. I had made it through the cancer journey. Life was good again. My heart was over-flowing with love and gratitude. My life had been blessed with so many beautiful moments along the rough road.

Two months later, I went back to work on May 12, starting part-time in order to slowly ease back into my job. It was good to be back. Seeing my co-workers and getting back into a routine was good, and life felt normal again.

SHARING MY CANCER STORY

Two years later, in August 2008, I attended Jack Canfield's Breakthrough to Success program in Scottsdale, Arizona, with Emily. At this seven-day workshop with four hundred attendees, I met a woman named Annabelle. She had just written her first book, and it was about being a breast cancer survivor. She told me she had some copies of her books for sale. I was very interested in reading it, so I bought one for myself and one for Emily. That night, I couldn't wait to start reading it.

The next day, I saw Annabelle again and told her how much I loved the book. I started to tell her of my experience with colon cancer, and she asked me to write my story.

I responded, "Write my story?"

"Yes, write me your story. I will put it in my next book," she said.

You could have knocked me over. Wow... I was asked to include my story in her book. I was so honored.

On November 3, 2008, I went to see Dr. Chhabra for my regular checkup and to have my blood work done. He was very pleased with my blood levels.

As an oncologist, Dr. Chhabra sees people every day who are sick and struggling to beat a disease that takes the lives of too many good people. Yet, here I was. Cancer-free, recovering from all my body had been through and happy to be alive. I had beaten the odds and life was good again. He was so very pleased to see that.

The doctor asked me if I had any questions for him. I didn't, but I told him I wanted to share a story with him.

RINGING THE BELL

When we're in the midst of things, we may not feel inspired or realize that we may be a role model to someone. But, whether we're healthy or sick, people we interact with every day are touched by us in subtle ways. A friendly smile or a kind word can brighten someone's day. How are you "showing up" in the world? How do you want to be remembered by others?

He was interested when I told him of meeting Annabelle and her asking me to write my story. I explained that I might need some of my medical records from him so my facts would be correct. Dr. Chhabra thought it was a great idea since my outcome was such a positive one. He felt there was a lot to be learned from my experience.

This conversation was the first time he ever told me that the average survival rate for Stage 4 colon cancer patients is eighteen months. I have to admit, I'm glad I hadn't known that earlier.

When you're fighting cancer, depression is a very real concern. Sometimes, you wonder if it's worth fighting and if you truly have the strength to get through it. If I had known the average survival rate, I may have given up during one of the more challenging times. Yet, as of this writing, it has been fifteen years since my colon surgery. The Lord has truly blessed me with his grace.

As I think back to that last little card Emily gave me in 2006 about sharing my story with others, little did I know that Annabelle would be the one to help me—a woman I didn't even know at the time. Annabelle's book was published in 2011 and was a collection of cancer stories from a variety of perspectives. Some stories were told by patients and others by family members. Yet, all were written to help support and encourage those facing cancer.

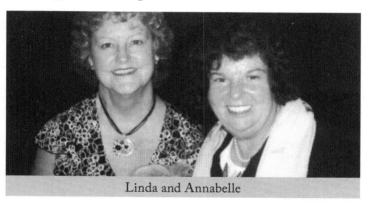
Linda and Annabelle

BEING OF SERVICE

In September 2008, I received our church newsletter in the mail. As I read through it, there was a request from the Prayer Shawl Ministry. They needed more people to join the group and knit prayer shawls. This group began meeting in 2003 and gets together once a month in a church member's home to knit with one another for ninety minutes.

The meeting begins with lighting a candle. Then, a prayer is read for those in need of comfort and for the knitters as they create their shawls. After these shawls are finished, they are taken to church and our pastor blesses them. After which, the shawls are ready to be given to those who are in need of comfort.

One of the members of the group named Sue made a shawl for me in 2005. She

RINGING THE BELL

Being treated for cancer, or helping a loved one who is undergoing treatment, may seem like something you'd prefer to forget when it's done. But this is a significant event in our life. It will change you in ways you can't even imagine. Embracing this time in your life with its many challenges will help you find peace and comfort. What beautiful memories do you want to carry with you five years from now?

knitted me a beautiful pink shawl and gave it to me during my colon cancer treatments.

To be of service and give back. Yes… I could do this. I called my friend Sue and told her I would like to join the group. So the next month, I attended the meeting. To this day, I am still a member and have hosted the group in my home.

During my colon cancer, I also enjoyed scrapbooking. When our daughter Emily brought me flowers and a note of encouragement for each chemo treatment, she took my picture with them for my scrapbook.

When I was cancer-free again, the idea eventually came to me to knit a shawl for the ministry the same color as the flowers I'd received for each of my treatments. The first flower was one yellow rose. So I made a yellow shawl. The second flowers were two purple irises. So I made a purple shawl. And so on.

Each page of my scrapbook shows the flowers, the shawl, the little card, and the picture of me. I enjoyed making the scrapbook, but most of all I still enjoy making prayer shawls for those in need of comfort, love and hope.

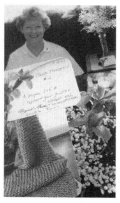

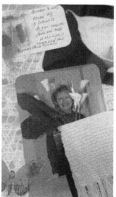

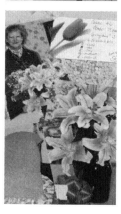

1 Yellow Rose
To represent your courage throughout.

2 Purple Irises
To represent your positive attitude and outlook.

3 Pink Baby Roses
To represent your inner strength.

4 Peach Baby Gerbera Daisies
To represent your sense of peace.

5 Calla Lilies
For your complete faith and trust in the Lord through all of this.

6 Birds of Paradise
Happy Halloween (Pooh)
For your glow of happiness and never-ending smile.

6 Sorbonne Lilies
½ way there:

C - Christ
H - Has
E - Every
M - Moment
O - Ordered

7 Yellow Tulips
For your always seeing the good in people and the positive.

8 Pink Chrysanthemums
Dear Mom,
For being the Best Mom any daughter could wish for. Thank you!

9 Matisse Roses

Dear Mom,

For keeping a smile on your face, having a sense of humor, and keeping focused on knowing the end is near... come on Disney.

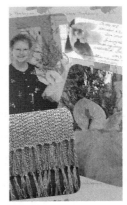

10 White Lilies

Dear Mom, For your perseverance!

11 Pink Hyacinths

Dear Mom,

For your acceptance of not "being in control" and letting Him take care of everything and trusting that it will all be taken care of... for you!

Love, Em

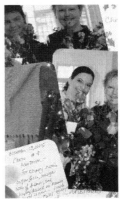

12 Assorted Pastel Roses

Dear Mom,

The last one. I know we thought this day would never get here. You have done amazing! You have gotten through these treatments so successfully and now are wanting to share your experience with others. You want to give others the hope, courage, encouragement and words of wisdom so they will be as successful as you have been.

I love you, Emily.

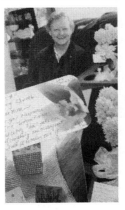

MESSAGE FROM PASTOR SUNGMU LEE

I have been Linda's pastor since July 1, 2014, serving at the First & Wesley United Methodist Church, where she has been an active member since 1960.

Linda has survived two serious illnesses: colon cancer and breast cancer. Although humans have made a great achievement with modern technology, we still have many other things we cannot control or explain. One of them is cancer, and I believe a spiritual approach to the disease is essential when we encounter the illness.

As a pastor and cancer survivor, I convinced Linda that God is with her, suffering with her, and giving her strength to overcome difficulties.

I believe that Linda's positive thinking has made a difference in her prognosis. She has had confidence and hope when there seemed no hope.

When I visit with a cancer patient in my congregation, I encourage them to have a positive attitude, which helps to overcome the illness.

I share Linda's case, letting other cancer patients know how important it is to be positive as we deal with cancer. As a pastor, I enjoy witnessing people like Linda overcoming difficulties through applying their Christian faith.

When I visited with Linda, I tried to console her. But when I came back home, I realized that I was also consoled by her positive thinking. Life is ups and downs, but it is up to us whether we are positive or not, regardless of our situations.

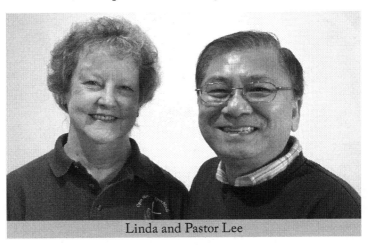

Linda and Pastor Lee

SUMMER DAYS

Today is a beautiful summer day. The cold days of winter are over. Daylight sticks around longer, and the air is fresh with smells of summer. It feels good to be outside in the warmth of the sun.

One of my favorite things to do is sit out on our back deck. Dennis and I spend a lot of time there. We are looking forward to enjoying picnics with family, walks along the beach with friends, and going out for ice cream cones in our 1964 Dodge Dart baby blue convertible.

This was in June 2016, and I was getting ready for work as usual. As I got dressed, I felt something in my left breast. *That's odd,* I thought. *I have never felt that before. I don't have any pain. But what is this? Dear God, I pray this is not cancer.* Of course, I was scared. I had already been through one bout with cancer. Thoughts of another cancer left me rattled. *This can't be happening again.*

I didn't say anything to Dennis at first. I didn't want to worry him. I said, "Goodbye" and "See you tonight," and off to work I went. All day I kept thinking of the possibility of breast cancer. Because of my past experience with colon cancer, I knew I had to find out.

I called my primary care physician, Dr. Laurence Knoll, and made an appointment for June 30, 2016. I didn't tell my doctor what I felt in my left breast. I wanted to see if he felt something without me saying anything to him. Sure enough, during the examination, he felt something as well.

We talked a while. He told me, "I have seen so much of this lately." Because I was going to my oncologist the following week for a checkup, we agreed to wait before making any appointments for tests.

Later that evening, after I got home from work, I told Dennis I might have another problem. We talked a while about the possibility of another cancer. This would mean our lives would turn upside down again.

A week later, on July 6, 2016, I went to see Dr. Chhabra for my post-colon cancer checkup. He asked me how I am doing. I pointed to my belly and said "I'm doing fine here, but I think I have a new problem here," pointing to my left breast. Dr. Chhabra immediately looked concerned. Examining me, he commented, "This is not normal." Right away, appointments were made to have a mammogram and ultrasound.

Although I had been having mammograms regularly, I had missed scheduling one in 2015. There had just been too many things going on in my life, and I let it slip

RINGING THE BELL

Fear of the unknown can make experiences so much harder. Your care providers are there, not just to treat your illness, but to answer your questions and help set your mind at ease. Don't be afraid to ask questions or to tell them how you are feeling. They may be able to provide answers or solutions that make this journey a bit easier for you. Are there questions you haven't asked yet that you wish you had? Go ask them now!

past, as so many women do. So this mammogram would be my first one in almost two years.

On July 11, 2016, I went for the tests. The results were not good. I was sent to Smilow Cancer Hospital for a biopsy three days later, on July 14, 2016.

I had never had a biopsy before. *What are they going to do*, I thought to myself. *Why is this happening?* All the old feelings of being scared came flooding back. I was grateful Dennis was with me.

Dr. Liane Philpotts, Chief of Breast Imaging at Smilow, explained the procedure to me. After she located the tumor, a small incision would be made to insert a needle to take several core samples that would be sent to a lab for analysis and then a marker would be put in. If surgery is needed, the marker shows the surgeon where to find the tumor. Dr. Philpotts took a biopsy on my left breast and the lymph nodes under my arm. While she did this, I had to hold my left arm over my head.

I kept thinking, *How much longer?* It felt like forever and my arm was falling asleep. Finally, after forty minutes, the procedure was over. Amen.

A few days later, I received the results. The biopsies came back positive for breast cancer. I had a very large lobular 8.5 cm tumor. I would need chemotherapy and surgery again. I also found out I would need radiation and hormone therapy.

All I could think about was my family. They went through the colon cancer with me, and this diagnosis meant another year with treatments, surgery and now radiation. There was so much ahead of us, for the second time.

FACING NEW FEELINGS

Once again, I would need a port before starting my chemo treatments, this time for breast cancer. This made August 24, 2016, another long and exhausting day. At Smilow Cancer Hospital, Dr. Jonathan Cardella inserted a port; this time on the right side of my chest, opposite where my last port had been. From there, I visited Dr. Chhabra at the oncology center for my first chemo treatment. I would receive the treatments once every three weeks for three months. They were each three to four hours long. The day after a treatment, I needed to go back to Dr. Chhabra for a Neulasta injection to help my white blood cell count.

After my second treatment, I started to lose my hair. It didn't thin like last time. It was actually falling out. I had been told this was going to

RINGING THE BELL

Different chemotherapy drugs have different side effects. And different people react to the drugs in their own unique ways. So, while it's helpful to know what the possible side effects may be and how to deal with them, don't assume the same thing will happen to you, especially when you hear someone else's horror story with this, that or the other treatment. The most important thing is, how are *you* doing?

happen, but until it does, you don't know how you are going to feel. I dreaded this part.

I knew it was time to do something after seeing so much hair in the drain after showering. Well... I asked my husband, "Would you buzz off my hair?" And, of course, he did. I held a towel in front of me and, as he buzzed my hair, he put the clippings on the towel.

This was very emotional for both of us. We had been married for forty-seven years at that point and have been through many of life's experiences together. This was one I was not prepared for. But Dennis is my soul mate and loves me even without my hair.

When he finished, I looked in the mirror. I had always taken a lot of pride in the way my hair looked, and now it was gone. This was a hard adjustment for me. I had no choice, though. I knew I must move forward and not let it get me down.

Since I knew I would lose my hair, I wanted to be pre-

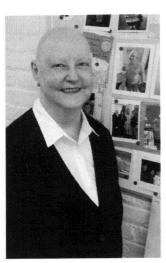

pared with a hat ahead of time. Wearing my colorful hats during my colon cancer treatment had boosted my spirit, and I had no doubt that it would again. So, a couple of weeks before chemo started, Dennis and I stopped in the Smilow Cancer Hospital Boutique to look at hats. I found a little pink one with a flower on it. Perfect... that was the one I wanted.

On chemo treatment days, my family came with me. One day, while I was having a treatment, Dennis and Emily said they needed to run an errand. When they came back, they were all smiles. Emily handed me a bag tied with a ribbon. In it, were six more little hats, all different colors... just what I wanted. Emily had picked out a nice assortment. Now I could match my hats with my outfits.

While I was receiving my treatment, we learned there was a 92-year-old woman having her last chemo treatment for breast cancer. Emily and I looked at each other, and she said, "We should give her a pink hat." We smiled at each other. Then Emily took the hat over to the woman, who received it with the biggest smile of gratitude on her face. We had made her day!

As the months went by and the holidays were nearing, I wanted a festive hat. We went shopping at Saxon and Kent Boutique, a local specialty shop for breast cancer patients, and found a red hat and a winter white one. These were great for Christmas and the winter season.

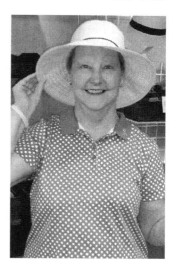

Every time I went to my doctor appointments, I wore a different color hat in a different style. Other patients begin to notice. I became known as "The Hat Lady." My hats brought smiles from many people and became fun to wear.

On November 16, 2016, I began a different chemo drug. This one was once a week for twelve weeks. Each treatment was two to three hours. Dr. Chhabra told me, "This drug will be easier for you."

I knew there would be some side effects, however, these were different. Sleeping became difficult. I just couldn't seem to settle myself at night. Listening to music by Jim Brickman helped a lot. Another side effect was nausea, like when I was pregnant with our daughters. I never expected to feel that way again. I was given pills to take care of that problem.

When I went through my chemotherapy treatments for both my cancers, food just didn't taste the same. My taste buds changed, as did my appetite. Everything tasted like cardboard. I knew I needed to eat to keep up my strength. One thing that helped me was to eat small meals. Sometimes just a quarter of a slice of toast was all I could eat. I discovered that if I ate every two hours, if only just a little, it made me feel better.

There were nights I couldn't sleep, I was so hungry. Many times, Dennis would warm up some soup for me in the middle of the night. Sometimes, I ate a little fruit cup or some applesauce, or a few peanut butter crackers with a glass of milk.

MESSAGE FROM LOU FRIEDMAN, PHYSICAL THERAPIST

I first met Linda in February 2017 at the Smilow Cancer Hospital. I saw her for a visit to take a baseline measurement of her arm before her mastectomy. We then began regular visits soon after when she came to me for physical therapy treatments for limitations she was having with her shoulder after her surgery for breast cancer. I learned that this was the second go-around for her, having had successful treatment for colon cancer previously.

Patients think we help them, and they benefit from our services and support. What they do not realize is that we as caregivers often receive as much, or more, than we give. This was the case with "Lovely Linda" and her inseparable sidekick and husband "Dynamic Dennis."

After her surgery, Linda came to me hardly able to move her left arm and concerned that this could impact her care by delaying her radiation from starting because she did not have enough range of motion to get into the proper position. The problem to solve was: how could we, as a team, get her arm moving well enough so she could proceed with her care as scheduled?

What evolved was a collaboration: Linda with her calm demeanor, warm smile, and lets-just-get-this-done attitude, Dennis with his helpful manner (not to mention helping hands), support from their two daughters, and guidance from me and the other caregivers.

Linda set her goal that she was not going to have any delay in her care because of her limitations. With that in mind, we continued as a team, modifying and adjusting her care as she progressed, until she achieved her goal of starting radiation.

This was a relief for Linda, but we were not done yet. Although she had enough range of motion to have her radiation, she still had pain and limitations that needed more work. She wanted to get back to her active lifestyle, which included among other things riding her bicycle, walking along the beach, and taking trips to see her two daughters who both lived out of state.

Each day that Linda came in for treatment, I received a smile and a thank you from her, as well as a handshake and thank you from Dennis. Soon the smile and thank you were replaced with a hug (from Linda, not Dennis).

There are several things that can be learned from this dynamic relationship.

Linda's success was a group effort and no one party was more important than the other. Without Dennis helping at home and without Linda having set goals and being determined to meet them, she may not have made the progress she did.

Dennis was willing to help in any way he could, no questions asked. It helped that he learned very quickly and is detail-oriented.

Dennis and Linda were tight. Their daughter Emily described them as inseparable. This, combined with the support from her two daughters, gave Linda the support and motivation to work through this difficult process.

Because of the nature of what we do in physical therapy, we spend a lot of time with patients and talk about many different topics. I am blessed repeatedly by people allowing me to be part of their journey in the battle we call "cancer," sharing their story, and allowing me to see past the shell and into the window of who they are. Invariably people change along this journey and come to understand and appreciate the important things in life. Although I think this was part of who Linda already was, I think this appreciation was compounded for her, having beaten colon cancer earlier and now dealing with her breast cancer.

Any caregiver who is willing to learn and listen has a great deal to gain. So for as many times as Linda thanked me, I must say a very big thank you to her for what I gained because I was a part of her journey.

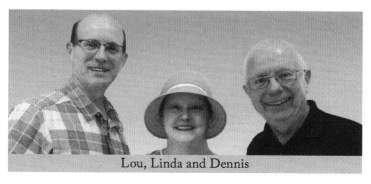

Lou, Linda and Dennis

THE MASTECTOMY

February 1, 2017, was my final chemotherapy treatment. I had made it through again. Praise the Lord! I was so grateful to have finished successfully. Now that the chemo treatments had ended, it was amazing how fast my taste buds came back. My appetite improved, and it was good to enjoy food again. I needed to rest for a few weeks before my surgery.

My energy level was getting stronger and life seemed better. It was now time to prepare myself for the surgery.

When Dennis buzzed off my hair in August 2016, I didn't go anywhere without my hat. Even around the house, I always wore my hat. All this time, the hardest thing for me was wanting to hide my bald head from my daughters. I didn't want them to see it.

One evening at the end of February, with my surgery two weeks away, I asked my daughters, "Girls, are you ready to see your mother without any hair?"

They looked at me surprised. "Yes, of course, Mom, if you want to show us."

I responded, "I think you need to be prepared how I look before surgery day." With that I took off my hat. I felt like

I was showing my private parts. They both said, "Mom… You look beautiful."

I then put my hat back on. It was time for a big family hug.

My breast surgeon Dr. Nina Horowitz explained to me I would need a total mastectomy because my tumor was very large and the cancer had spread to the neighboring lymph nodes. She was also the one who had told me that it is very common to get lymphedema after surgery when lymph nodes are being removed, and who sent me to see Lou Friedman to take measurements of my arm as a baseline prior to surgery.

RINGING THE BELL

Each of us have different experiences with loss as we go along this journey. Some losses are physical, others are emotional. Some are temporary, and others are more permanent. Regardless of the loss you experience, allow yourself to grieve. No matter how big or small the loss is, you have the right to grieve it in your own way and your own time. Don't deny yourself that right.

March 7, 2017, the day of my surgery, came quickly enough. Dennis, Jen, Emily and I headed to the hospital. We were ready to get this over with. They stayed in the waiting room while I had the surgery to remove my left breast and sixteen more lymph nodes (of which five were cancerous this time). All went well with the surgery, and I only needed to stay one night in the hospital. Both Jen and Emily spent the night with me. I was so glad they were there. They provided such comfort to me.

For some reason, I felt all right about losing my breast. I can't explain it. I felt worse when I had the drain for my colon cancer. Maybe because I couldn't see what was going on inside of me then. With the breast, I can see. Yes, my body looks different, but I'm okay with it. The main thing for me is the cancer is gone. I will recover and life will be good again.

The next day, Dennis arrived to pick us up. The girls and I were ready to go home. The nurse came to my room with instructions, and I was discharged from the hospital.

With a big sigh, I knew I was going home. When I arrived there, a huge bouquet of flowers greeted me. It was from all of my cousins, my sister and my nieces. I am so blessed by the love of my family.

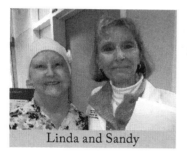
Linda and Sandy

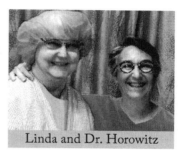
Linda and Dr. Horowitz

Message from Lynore Aaron, Certified Fitter

The Boutique at Smilow Cancer Hospital is a warm and safe environment for patients and guests. Situated right off the main entrance, it is visible to all. It offers beautiful retail items as well as head coverings, skin care and comfortable clothing for patients going through treatment. It also is where I am located. As the certified fitter for mastectomies and lymphedemas, I see both women and men in the back of the Boutique. This makes the Boutique a true jewel.

I remember the day I met Linda. She came in to be fitted with post-surgical camisoles to wear after her upcoming mastectomy. She was with her husband Dennis and their two daughters, Jen and Emily. She was wearing a soft pink head cap, which made her face light up.

The two girls came into the fitting room with Linda. The three were a bit apprehensive about the unknown. I spent time answering questions and explaining that she would return to see me in four to six weeks to be fitted with bras and a prosthesis.

I was taken with the two girls and their concern and love for their mother. This was truly a family that would make the journey together. They were the support team Linda would need. They left that appointment smiling and hugging.

Within two weeks, Linda was back to see me. Again, she was accompanied by Jen and Emily. Dennis had to patiently wait out front! Linda told me she needed a non-weighted prosthesis and soft bra because she was out and about. She had places to go and things to do—she was already going to church and taking walks. This woman was going to show the world that cancer was not going to take over her life.

She was thrilled to have a left breast again! And again, I was taken with her beautiful smile and kind, soft nature.

A few months later, on June 21, 2017, the big day came for the real prosthesis and mastectomy bras. We had fun and laughed a lot as I showed them a selection of bras and prostheses. Linda had no trouble making up her mind. She chose a very comfortable bra with great support and then selected a lightweight prosthesis. She looked awesome! She went out to show off her new body to Dennis, and he hugged and kissed her.

Two months later, Linda returned. This time, it was to be measured and fitted with a compression sleeve and glove for her left arm and hand. She had developed lymphedema and was being treated by Lou Friedman. She again accepted this with grace and dignity. She was not frightened; she smiled and said she would do whatever it took to get back out and be active again.

And she did. I now see her twice a year for fittings. She comes in with interesting stories of her trips to Cape Cod, her long walks, and her visits with the two girls. I always look forward to seeing her. She never fails to have a big smile on her face and a bear hug for me.

I feel so fortunate to be in my profession. I am able to enjoy the journey with each woman, from before surgery to after, and to see the smiles on their faces as I fit them with bras and prostheses. There is nothing more fulfilling than watching a woman's face light up as she takes her first look in the mirror and exclaims she feels "whole again." I am the one who receives the gift of giving.

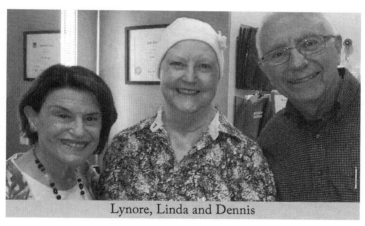

Lynore, Linda and Dennis

RADIATION ONCOLOGY

I made it through chemotherapy and surgery twice. But, now I faced a new experience. It was time to talk with Dr. Suzanne Evans about radiation oncology. Since the chemotherapy did not shrink the entire tumor and I still had some cancer in the lymph nodes at the time of my surgery, I had to have radiation for six weeks.

On April 5, 2017, I went for a CT scan with Dr. Evans at Smilow Cancer Hospital. This scan was used to establish my radiation treatment plan. Since it was a new experience for me, I was a little nervous. But Dr. Evans and all of the nurses were so kind to me. They walked me through the setup process and explained everything as we went along.

RINGING THE BELL

There will be times when your body needs a rest or your treatment plan needs adjusting to accommodate how you're feeling. And that's okay! Your doctor has studied long and hard to discover the right plan for each of their patients. Let your care providers know when something isn't working for you so they can make things as easy as possible for you.

During the CT scan, I needed to hold my breath. Each deep breath helps the nurses adjust the beams according to the doctor's orders. But I was having a hard time getting the timing right. When I finally got it right, I found out that my treatment plan would take two weeks to prepare.

Before leaving, another doctor, Dr. Chris Corso, sat with us. He happened to be walking past us when we were getting ready to leave, and he saw I was very upset. He asked if he could be of some help and that's when he joined us.

Dennis, Jen and Emily had many questions. Honestly, I was too overwhelmed to think of any. Dr. Corso spent a lot of time answering their questions and explaining in detail what the nurses had said. It was so much for all of us to take in.

On April 17, 2017, my treatment plan was ready. We took a test run to be sure everything was lined up correctly. But I had a problem. I was supposed to take deep breaths and hold my breath, just as I did during the setup process two weeks earlier. I tried and tried, but just couldn't get it right.

Dr. Evans changed my treatment plan to "normal breathing" and told me, "This will make it easier for you." She needed another week to set up the new plan for me.

I must say I was very discouraged with myself. But I needed to realize everyone is different and not everyone has the same treatment plan.

On April 24, 2017, I went for another test run. This time there were no deep breaths, just normal breathing. It went so well. All I needed to do was lay very still and put my arms in some arm rests. All of the nurses were great—Kathy, Nancy and another Kathy. They made sure my body was positioned perfectly.

The next day, it was time for my first live radiation treatment. It went well, and I felt so much happier with myself. My treatments were scheduled for every weekday for six weeks. Before each treatment, I needed to check in at the front desk. As the days went by, I was getting to know the girls at the front desk, and they always greeted me with a smile—Tracy, Lisa and Cheryl.

After I checked in, I went to a changing room and then waited in a waiting room until it was my turn. While I waited, I got to know some of the other patients. It was good to talk with them as we shared our experiences with each other.

Once a week, I met with the clinical nurses to follow up on how the previous week of treatments went. As the weeks went by, the treatment area became red. I was given Eucerin cream, which helped to keep my skin hydrated and soft.

Nancy, who was one of my nurses, told me to use saline solution as well. She said it would help with the healing of my skin.

My care providers called my sixth week of radiation "the boost." This focused on the incision area. My tumor had been very large, and we wanted to be sure no cancer cells remained. The boost burned my skin. Using the saline solution three times a day was the most soothing remedy I found and was very helpful to me. All along the way, the doctors and nurses made me feel safe and comfortable.

June 7, 2017, was my last radiation treatment. Yeah! I made it! Amen. My husband and daughters were always

RINGING THE BELL

When you're healthy, "normal" may seem boring. However, when you're ill, every day takes on a whole new meaning, and no event is too big or too small to celebrate. What are you going to celebrate today?

with me. I never felt alone. This was the day I got to hit the gong.

It's a pretty cool thing when the radiation department announces your last day of treatment. There is a gong on the wall. They'll say something like, "We have a graduate today." When it was my turn, they announced my name and handed me the rubber mallet. I hit the gong and a loud sound was heard by all. Everyone clapped their hands for me and smiled. I felt so happy and such a sense of relief.

A full year had passed, and I was cancer-free once again. Thank you, God!

Radiation was over, but I still had two more things I needed to do. The first was to start taking a hormone therapy pill. So, on June 27, 2017, I went back to Dr. Chhabra, and he gave me a prescription for letrozole. I will take one tablet each day for five years.

The second thing I needed to do was to have a bone density test. The results showed I have pre-osteoporosis. Because of this and the effects of the letrozole, I needed to have an infusion of zoledronic acid every twelve weeks to keep my bones strong. This was administered at the oncology center, taking thirty minutes each time, and will continue for five years as well.

Throughout all of this, my body has done very well. My hair started to grow back in February 2017 and by the fall of 2017 it was long enough to put curlers in.

I am so blessed to recover from cancer a second time. Along the way, I met so many wonderful people. With their caring words of encouragement, I became a stronger person. I learned more about myself than I ever knew before.

No matter what your particular journey entails, there will be beauty in it. May my story bring you hope as you make your own journey and remind you that you are not alone. Blessings to you, dear reader.

MESSAGE FROM DR. SUZANNE EVANS, RADIATION ONCOLOGIST

I am a radiation oncologist at Smilow Cancer Hospital at Yale-New Haven who specializes in breast cancer. It's a profession that's not well known to most patients and also not known to some physicians! It's not something most people spend time on during medical school. Just as medical oncologists prescribe chemotherapy to treat cancer, we prescribe radiation to treat cancer. We work independently from, but closely with, surgeons and medical oncologists as part of a multidisciplinary cancer team. Radiation is a powerful x-ray that is safe and effective for cancer treatment.

The side effects of radiation are all very localized, and most patients don't lose their hair or get nauseous from radiation. They are not typically radioactive, either. Treatments are usually given once a day for as short as two weeks or as many as nine. I meet with patients to decide whether radiation would help with the management of their cancer, weekly during treatment, and in the months (or years) following it.

For breast cancer, radiation has been shown to improve survival after a mastectomy when lymph nodes are involved, as well as when a lumpectomy is used and the breast is preserved. This means radiation is used for a lot of women following a breast cancer diagnosis!

I think what helps people get through this difficult diagnosis is to keep a positive attitude. Both patients and doctors do their best to cure the cancer with minimal side effects. When I design a radiation treatment plan for a patient, goals 1 through 10 are always to cure the cancer, if it is curable. I am grateful that with modern radiation treatment, I get to have parallel goals—curing the cancer and leaving as few "footprints" on the patient as possible. I always am conscious of how I can design the radiation plan in such a way as to minimize the risks of future side effects, not just current ones.

I think patients who face this difficult diagnosis should remember that cure rates for cancer are improving greatly. Don't be afraid to ask what your prognosis is once all of the appropriate tests have been performed. But keep in mind that you are not a statistic! Doctors can never be certain what any individual's course may be and, even if the outlook is not what you hope for, there's no reason why you cannot be the outlier and do better than anyone expects. If you have fire and fight in you, your journey will reflect that!

I want my patients to feel free to ask questions, even questions they feel might be silly. I encourage second opinions if patients desire them. However, I do feel it is important for patients to seek such opinions from reputable sources. Do your research. As a radiation oncologist who specializes in breast cancer, with 95% of my practice comprised of breast cancer, it will come as no surprise to you that I feel that those of us who specialize in one or just a few disease sites provide care that's a cut above people who are generalists and treat everything. (I'm probably biased!) There are exceptions to every rule, of course. But find out what your caregiver's practice is like. Ultimately, the most important thing is that you trust them with your life. If you don't feel right, then keep up your search until you find the right fit.

My favorite thing about being a radiation oncologist is I have the nicest patients! I treat mostly women, so they are moms, daughters, granddaughters, sisters, aunts, teachers, coaches, CEOs, doctors, scientists, small business owners, chefs… You name it. At this point, I know most of their concerns, and I love being able to help them through this tough time.

I love how logical radiation is. If you respect these rules, you can expect this likelihood of complications and success. I love the anatomy, and I love designing a plan and making it the best I possibly can. It's very satisfying to know you are part of someone's care.

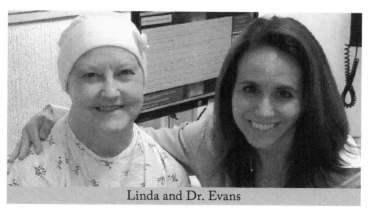

Linda and Dr. Evans

THE HEALING GARDEN

I would like to share an idea I had one day when I was at the Smilow Cancer Hospital. On this day, I was there for a test. Dennis, Jen and Emily were with me when we heard there was a healing garden on the 7th floor. So after I finished my test, we decided to go see this garden.

It was on the roof of the hospital. As you enter the garden, there is a path around it with benches, trees, bushes, flowers and a stream of water. It was a beautiful July day. Many family members and patients were walking around and some were sitting on the benches just enjoying the sun, fresh air and being out of the hospital; so peaceful, calming and, of course, healing.

On our way home, I kept thinking of the healing garden and how peaceful I felt there. Our backyard is like a little park. I enjoy spending time out there. It is much like the healing garden. But what about when the cold weather starts and winter comes?

On the left side of our house, we have a small heated room. Before, we used it as an office, but now it was just used for storage. The idea came to mind, "Let's clear it out and make it into a healing room." So I shared the idea with my family.

Dennis and the girls thought this was a great idea. That afternoon, they began to clear out the room, which has many windows, making it nice and sunny. It also has a glass sliding door so you can look out into the backyard to watch the birds, squirrels and visiting cats pass through the yard while watching the change of the seasons.

The next day, we shopped for new sheer curtains and hung them up. The transformation had begun; it was open, bright, and peaceful with a feeling of healing. Just what I wanted.

RINGING THE BELL

What brings you peace? Do you enjoy the outdoors? Being with people? Sitting by a roaring fire? Listening to music? Make a list of those things you enjoy the most and find a way to bring them into your life regularly.

I have spent so much time in this room since then. It truly is a healing place for me. Some people don't have a spare room like I do. Maybe a small table could be set up with inspirational stones, books, words or pictures. Cards can be taped to a door. I received many encouraging cards and hung mine on the curtains.

My treatments were finished in June 2017, yet we still continue to use this room. Dennis and I start our day in it. We have our breakfast together there and plan our day. Even our two cats, Boston and Sweet Pea, want to be in there too. They love to watch the birds. This room has brought us all so much joy.

THE SURPRISE

One of my favorite music artists is Jim Brickman. He is a songwriter and solo piano player. I have been listening to his music for several years now. I not only listened to Jim's music at home, but also when I was working in the nursing home before I retired. His music is calming and uplifting, and it played a big part in my recovery from breast cancer.

I have seen Jim in concert three times. If you ever have an opportunity to go see him, you won't be disappointed. It truly is a wonderful experience. In December 2017, Dennis and I went to see Jim at The Turning Stone Casino in upstate New York. Our daughter Emily and our son-in-law Ed met us there for dinner before the concert. Our friends, Teresa and Bill, joined us as well.

There are so many nice places to eat in the casino. We have a favorite Italian restaurant. Ed made reservations for us and, when we arrived, we were seated right away. Since it was Christmas-time, the restaurant was beautifully decorated.

During dinner, Emily, Ed, Teresa and Bill had Christmas gifts for us. There was one gift in particular that made them all smile. Dennis and I looked at each other. What could this be? As we opened a card, we found VIP tickets inside to a Meet and Greet with Jim Brickman. Oh my goodness… What a moment of pure *joy*.

So after dinner and before the concert, we all waited our turn to see Jim. Emily had brought him a t-shirt we had made for friends and family that said "Team Linda." As we waited, our excitement built. Finally, our turn arrived, and Jim greeted us with a warm smile.

Emily told him I was a breast cancer survivor and that we had a gift for him. The back of the t-shirt listed all the things that make me happy. At the very top was the name "Jim Brickman." She explained to him how much his music helped me while I was going through my chemotherapy, surgery and radiation treatments. She told him, "My mom listens to your music all the time."

I then thanked him for his gift of music and told him what a comfort it was to me—how it made me feel peaceful and calm. I told him I even listen to his music throughout the night. Meeting Jim was so special to me. He gave us all a hug and thanked us for coming. What a special Christmas gift.

It was now time for the concert and to find our seats. Teresa had ordered the tickets. As the usher led us to our seats, we kept walking closer and closer to the stage. Another great surprise. We were seated in the second row from the stage… directly facing Jim. Another moment of *joy*. Fittingly, the name of the concert was "A Joyful Christmas." It truly was.

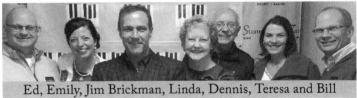

Ed, Emily, Jim Brickman, Linda, Dennis, Teresa and Bill

MESSAGE FROM EMILY ALBERTS, LINDA'S DAUGHTER

We are "Team Linda," formed to support one special woman—Linda Kopec—my mom. The group originated in August 2016, soon after Mom was diagnosed with breast cancer. We chose to gather together to recognize and appreciate the many people who rose to the occasion during this challenging time—friends and family, doctors, nurses and other medical professionals, angels among us each and every day in so many ways.

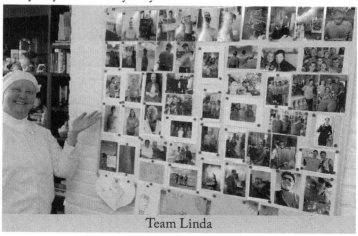

Team Linda

The seed for our team was planted by a good friend of the family named Debbie, never realizing just how large the team would become. (As of July 2020, it was 175 people in all.) We are humbled by the love, support and kindness we were surrounded with throughout this process. If you are going through a challenging time, I highly recommend you form a team too. It makes all the difference in the world.

These are people who are skilled, knowledgeable, dedicated, compassionate, interested, thoughtful and right there when you need a hand, a shoulder, an ear or some words of wisdom and guidance. Each person on the team is unique and special. Each giving something that only they can give. Each connected to a healing circle—the healing circle of love.

Cancer can be a scary word. However, when you have a team supporting you, somehow the feeling of being scared transforms into confidence, comfort and safety. Every step of the way, we felt supported and cared for. That's a gift we can never repay to those who are on our team.

RACE FOR THE CURE

The Susan G. Komen Race for the Cure is an education and fundraising event for breast cancer. This 5K run benefits those who have been diagnosed with breast cancer and celebrates survivors. It is filled with courage, bravery, strength, connections, positivity, recognition, appreciation and awareness.

My friend Nicole and I completed this race about ten years ago as runners. We were very much into athletics at that time. This time, it was different. On May 19, 2018, we walked with Nicole's mom and dad, Toni and Wayne, as well as my mom and dad.

The day arrived complete with raindrops and umbrellas, puddles and rain jackets. There were smiles and pink—lots and lots of pink. Registration began at 8:00 a.m. The six of us wore smiles from ear to ear, excited to participate in this event together. One team. One family. One mission.

We stayed together the entire journey. The number in attendance was low due to the rain, cold and wind. For some reason, the rain simply fueled us.

Many times, I told my mom, "If at any point you want to stop or not do this, just say so." The response from my mom, as well as the others, was, "I'm not giving up." This was her motto for pretty much the entire two years prior as she went through treatments (port placement, chemotherapy, surgery, radiation, wound care and hormone therapy). She simply never gave up. Quitting was simply not an option.

I remember being amazed at how brave, how strong, how determined, and how matter-of-fact she was throughout. But come to think of it, that is pretty much how she has always been. She has always lived a life of "I'm not giving up, and I will do what it takes." My dad shares the same positive attitude. So together, nothing could stop them, and nothing will ever stop them. They are unstoppable.

The survivor parade started at 8:30 a.m. I felt it was important to participate in this. So, Mom, Dad and I marched in the parade, umbrellas and all, with smiles and rain gear. The bagpipes began their symphony of music as the sea of pink trailed behind them, walking in formation to the stage where the opening ceremonies were to take place.

Just as we began to walk, Mom and I arm-in-arm, our umbrella flipped inside out. I suddenly heard a sweet voice say, "Here, take mine. Use this one. Come, let's walk. I'll walk with you." A kind young lady proceeded to hold the umbrella over us and walk right by our side. Meanwhile, there is my dad, right behind us, taking the umbrella and fixing it. That is how my dad has always been—"a fixer"—one who takes care of things, especially for his wife and his girls (me and my sister Jen). How grateful we are. How spoiled with love.

The young woman asked, "So, what's your story?" As she continues to walk with us, shielding us from the wet and cold rain, we tell her about Mom being diagnosed with breast cancer. She responds, "I was diagnosed years ago too." We were instantly connected forever through vulnerability, kindness and bravery; a bond forged of steel. Tears began to well up in our eyes.

Together, we walked. Together, we cared. Together, we were one.

The woman's name? Holly. Simply another person on Team Linda—right there when we needed someone. That is how this whole journey has been. Right when we needed someone, an angel showed up to lend a hand, tell a story, make us laugh, make us cry (tears of joy or appreciation), or offer a word of encouragement.

The walk began at 10:15 a.m. There were individual umbrellas for Wayne, Toni, Mom and Dad. But Nicole and I? We chose to share one as we walked arm-in-arm for portions of the walk. Side-by-side, we walked with our parents a short distance behind us.

We told stories along the way, remembering, reflecting and reminiscing. We smiled, laughed and cried. We were grateful and appreciative the entire 3.1 miles. We felt inspired to set new goals, something we always do. Setting the goal of completing the Race for the Cure allowed us to connect with one another and encourage one another, like we always do. Some people wait to celebrate at the completion of a goal. Yet, we choose to celebrate the moments along the way.

One hour and eight minutes later, Team Linda crossed the finish line. Nicole and I first, followed by Wayne, Toni, Mom and Dad. "Number 66, Linda Kopec, a survivor, crossing the finish line right now. Congratulations, Linda! We have been waiting for you!"

Smiles beamed from my mom and dad as well as Wayne and Toni. Tears of gratitude and appreciation welled up in my eyes. Hugs were exchanged among each of us along with a "We did it! Congratulations!"

This race signified so much. It was a challenging goal that called us to review and reflect upon all that had happened over the years. Ultimately, it became a celebration of all of the little moments that got us to where we are.

There was nothing that could have gotten us down on this day. We chose to respond with happiness, appreciation, joy, confidence and celebration, and we succeeded... together. We are Team Linda. We are stronger together, and we are braver because of one another.

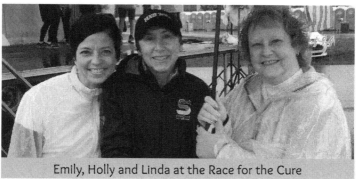

Emily, Holly and Linda at the Race for the Cure

Final Thoughts

As we go through this journey called "life," things happen unexpectedly, both good and bad. I think celebrating the good things in life is so important. Celebrating brings us joy and a sense of well-being.

When bad things happen, we aren't always prepared. Sometimes, we don't know how to handle or accept it. These are the times when we must be strong. We need to grow in faith and believe things will turn out alright. We will overcome whatever problem we are facing.

Time has passed, and I am still cancer-free, for which I'm grateful. But life has kept me on my toes.

On a winter day in March 2020, when the Covid-19 pandemic had just started, I got up as usual and went downstairs to get things ready for breakfast. Typically, I would go back upstairs after our meal to shower and get dressed. But this day, I started down the stairs to the cellar. I needed to get something from the downstairs refrigerator.

I was wearing slippers, but I always wear my slippers around the house without any problems. This day was different though. For some reason, my foot slipped on the tread and down the stairs I went, with my left leg trapped under my right one.

I sat a minute from the shock and then pulled my leg out from under me only to see my foot dangling. *Oh no!* I thought. *I can't fix this!*

I called Dennis, who was at the other end of the house. He came right away. Taking one look at my foot, he said, "I need to make a phone call. I'll be right back."

So, there I sat in a short summer nighty, undies and my glasses.

Dennis had no sooner come back from making the phone call, when the ambulance arrived. The paramedics wrapped my leg in a large towel and medical tape to form a soft cast and then lifted me onto a stretcher.

As I was wheeled out to the ambulance, Dennis handed me my cell phone and said he would follow in his car to the hospital.

When I was wheeled into the emergency room, Dennis was not allowed in; because of Covid-19, only patients could enter the hospital.

Lucky for me, I had my cell phone. Dennis texted me that he would wait in the parking lot. So there I was, in pain and all alone. I needed to have x-rays and a CT scan. It turned out I had broken two bones, the tibia and the fibula, and I was going to need surgery, which was scheduled for the next morning.

I texted Dennis about the surgery and told him he should go home. After he got there, he called our daughters to let them know what happened.

My surgery took two and a half hours. Rods and screws were put in my leg, and all went well. I was still in pain but not as bad as it had been after the fall.

The next day, a physical therapist came to my room to get me up and walking with a walker. She said not to put my full weight on the leg.

I didn't do too well, at first. I could only take three steps because of the pain. But then she told me that if I could walk to the hall and back to my bed, I could go home tomorrow. That's all I needed to hear. I was determined and thought, *I'm going home.*

The next day, when she came back to my room, I walked to the hall and back to my bed. She said, "Good job! You can go home now." So, I texted Dennis I was coming home.

Because of the pandemic, I didn't want Dennis to come back to the hospital to pick me up. I told the nurse I would go home by the wheelchair transportation service.

She asked me, "You know that will cost you $75?"

I said, "I don't care. I don't want my husband near the hospital with this virus around."

To my surprise, a little after I got home, our daughters came to visit. They both stayed with us for three weeks. Emily is a physical therapist and showed me exercises to help with the healing and walking with the walker. Jen helped with moving things from my bedroom upstairs to the bedroom downstairs. The girls helped with washing clothes, sheets, cooking, shopping, and anything that came up that we needed help with.

Dennis became my doctor at home. I needed a blood thinner so I didn't get clots in my leg. It had to be administered by a needle and was to be given in my belly every day for five weeks. We called it "the dreaded needle."

It was six months before I could walk without the walker. Once the surgeon saw I could get around without it, he said

I could start walking on my own. That's all I wanted to hear. Nine months have passed since I broke my leg, and I am now pretty much back to normal.

Even though this experience was different from my cancers, there are things that remain the same... The gifts and lessons I learned before still apply.

> *I am grateful*
> for my doctor,
> who put me back to together.
>
> *I am grateful*
> for my family,
> who took care of all my needs.
>
> *I had to practice acceptance*
> while waiting for healing
> to take place in my broken bones.
>
> *I persevered*
> with my exercises
> so I could walk again.

There will be times when life is hard and times when things seem easier. But practicing gratitude, acceptance and perseverance makes all the difference in our perception.

Right now, my life is good once more. But I know that I can rely on these three gifts to see me through no matter what comes my way.

And so, my dear reader, I hope that as you practice these lessons in your own life journey, you will reach a point of being able to say, "My life is good once more" too.

God bless!

AFTERWORD

As Linda Kopec's husband, I wonder what I could possibly add to such a sincere, heartfelt book as the one my wife has so lovingly written. As a caregiver to Linda during her experiences with cancer, all I could really do was be there for her. I hope that I was present for Linda enough to help her feel safe and loved. When you think about it, that's the best thing we can do.

My wife never complains about anything. Even after fifty years of marriage, I'm still trying to figure out how I got so lucky. Over the years, we have faced many problems together, both big and small. I must admit, cancer has been our biggest challenge yet. There were so many feelings to deal with.

I will never forget the first visit to Smilow Cancer Hospital. Seeing the numbers of people, visibly not well, coming and going for treatment. It made me feel both fearful and hopeful at the same time.

If you are a caregiver, know that your role can make a huge difference for the patient, and surprisingly maybe for yourself. There were many things Linda was not able to do without assistance, and I was glad I could help her.

Perhaps more importantly, I imagine the journey through cancer can be very lonely. I was happy to know that my presence could provide some level of comfort. It's the little things that make a big difference. I had to constantly remind myself of this, and still do.

We are a family who looks out for each other. If one of us needs help, we are all ready to pitch in—ready to do everything we can, with no limits. It is with this insight that I mention that the well-being of the caregiver is also important. Remember to take care of yourself, so you can care for your loved one.

Linda inspires me in so many ways. Curiously enough, I don't think she even knows that she does.

Linda, I love you so much. Thank you. Sign me up for another fifty years.

— *Dennis Kopec*

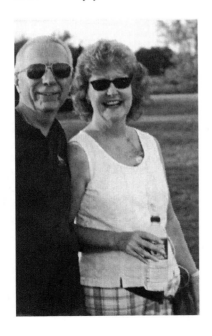

Thank you for reading *Cancer Gifts*.
If you've enjoyed reading this book, please leave a review
on your favorite review site. It helps me reach more readers
who may benefit from the information provided herein.

Acknowledgments

It is with deep appreciation that I express my gratitude to all my medical providers, family and friends. Without you, I would not be writing this book.

Dr. Ikekpeazu, you have been with me since the start of my colon cancer diagnosis. Once you saw the tests results, you knew just what needed to be done. The surgery took a long time since there was a lot going on inside of me. Yet, all the necessary procedures were completed. You saved my life, and I will be forever grateful.

Dr. Chhabra, we have been on a cancer journey together since 2005. You took care of me when I had my colon cancer. Then, in 2016, as soon as you saw I had a problem with my breast, you took action and set up appointments for tests right away. Once my diagnosis was confirmed, chemotherapy dates were set up. Throughout these years, we have had a special patient-doctor bond. Thank you from a grateful heart.

Sandy Hurd, we will always be grateful for all the hours you spent on the phone with us. With your wealth of knowledge, you were able to answer all of our questions. It was a difficult time, and you gave us all the time we needed. Some decisions were hard to make, but with your kind and gentle guidance, we were able to make them. Thank you from grateful hearts.

Lou Friedman, because of you, I have come so far with my range of motion since February 2017. After surgery, it was so hard for me to move my left arm. But with your expertise in physical therapy, I was able to begin to move my arm more, with less pain. You showed Dennis what he could do at home to help me. You also helped Jen understand what she could do for me through massage therapy. You answered many questions Emily had. As time went on, we all became good friends. Thank you for all you did to help us. This was truly a team effort.

Dr. Horowitz, when I learned of my breast cancer, I had no idea of which surgeon to go to. At the time, I was working at a nursing home and a co-worker told me about your skill in breast cancer treatment. She highly recommended you to perform my surgery. My family and I met you on August 1, 2016. You made us all feel so at ease. You answered all our questions. On surgery day, you wore your Team Linda shirt and we all laughed together. My co-worker was right… You are the *best*. Thank you, thank you, for taking such good care of me.

Dr. Kopel, months after my colon cancer surgery, you assured me Dr. Ikekpeazu had made best choices for my situation and that you were impressed with his work. These words made me feel so blessed to have the best surgeon possible.

Dr. Evans, radiation was a new experience for me. Six weeks seemed like a long time. My family and I had so many questions. You took the time to answer them right from Day One. Each person is different, and you designed a treatment plan that was right for me. I knew I would get through this just as I had done with chemotherapy and surgery. Thank you for always making me feel safe.

Lynore, the kind of work you do is very personal. After surgery, our bodies look very different. It can be embarrassing for others to see. Having a mastectomy is one of those times. You have a special gift of making people feel relaxed, including me. You were with me every step of the way, from when I needed a post-surgical camisole to a non-weighted prosthesis and soft bra, and then to the real prosthesis and mastectomy bra. I went from feeling broken to feeling whole again. Through this process, we have developed a special bond, one woman to another. There are not enough words to express my gratitude. You are very special to me. Love to you.

Pastor Lee, thank you for all your visits to my house. We shared our cancer stories together, talked of being positive each day, and shared our Christian faith and our trust in the Lord. I always felt the greatest gift given to me by my mother was faith. Now, sharing my faith with you has been a blessing. God bless.

Team Linda, thank you all so much for your love and support. I received so many get-well cards, text messages, emails, phone calls, food deliveries, bouquets (both of flowers and fruit), and other gifts. Every one of you made a huge difference in my recovery. I am so grateful for all of you.

Church family, as soon as it was announced I had cancer, you began praying for me every day. Pastor Yost came to visit me when I had my colon cancer. Later, Pastor Lee came to visit during my breast cancer treatments. Every week, I received so many cards. They brought me so much joy and encouragement. By the grace of God, I have been blessed twice.

Word Weavers Berkshires, you are such a special group of gifted writers. Writing has never been my strength, but you welcomed me into the group. With your help, I began to learn. Every month, the words started to come together and now I am so excited to say "my book is ready to bring hope."

Tara Alemany and Mark Gerber from Emerald Lake Books, working with the two of you to publish my book has been a true pleasure. I have learned so much. As you know, I am a little technically challenged, but you were so patient with me. We just went step-by-step, and it all came together so nicely. This book was a dream of mine for many years and now it is reality. My goal has been reached, and my book is ready to bring hope, love and support to everyone whose lives are touched by cancer. My heart is filled with gratitude. Thank you both so much for everything.

My sister Joan and niece Amy, during my colon cancer treatments, you came to my house nearly every day to see if I needed help with anything. Many times, you would pick me up and we would go out for lunch together. Some days, we took walks at the beach or went shopping. But, most importantly, you took me to my doctor's appointments. Thank you both so much.

Jen, my massage-therapist daughter. How can I thank you for all the massages? You helped my body rest and relax. Any pain or discomfort I had, your skilled hands knew just how to fix. You made so many trips from Massachusetts to Connecticut to be with me. No words can thank you enough for all you did. I am so grateful.

Emily, you became my secretary, made all of the phone calls (especially for medical follow-ups). You were the spokes-person for the family. You asked many questions so we all understood my plan of treatment and what to expect as time went on. You became my shopper when I needed clothes, shoes and other items since I didn't want to be around crowds and pick up any germs. You also drove a long way to be with me, from upstate New York to coastal Connecticut. Saying thank you is not enough. I am at a loss for words and so grateful for you.

Dennis, my loving husband of over fifty years, we have been through the sickness and health part of our marriage twice now. Without you by my side, I would not have done as well. You took care of all my needs, from doing the food shopping, taking me to my appointments, running the errands, cleaning dishes, washing clothes, and so many more things. I thank you for all you did to help make my recovery successful. We have been blessed with a beautiful life together.

ABOUT THE AUTHOR

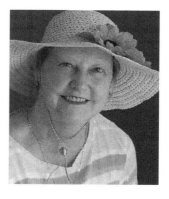

Linda Kopec was a payroll bookkeeper for over twenty years. After surviving both colon cancer and breast cancer, she decided it was time to retire and write her inspiring story of surviving cancer twice.

While writing was not Linda's natural strength, she was determined to learn how to do it well. It was important to her to share her stories of survival to encourage others, and it pleases her that *Cancer Gifts: Lessons in Gratitude, Acceptance and Perseverance* is ready to bring hope, love and support to all who read it.

Linda now works at home with her husband Dennis. They have an accounting business called Sea Bluff Accounting, LLC.

Linda and Dennis have been married for over fifty years and make their home in West Haven, Connecticut. They have two grown daughters, who live out of state.

If you're interested in having Linda come speak to your group or organization, either online or in person, you can contact her at emeraldlakebooks.com/kopec.

For more great books, please visit us at
emeraldlakebooks.com.

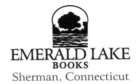

EMERALD LAKE
BOOKS
Sherman, Connecticut